BACTERIOLOGY PRIMER IN AIR CONTAMINATION CONTROL

Bacteriology Primer
in
Air Contamination
Control

BY V. VICTOR KINGSLEY

School of Hygiene
University of Toronto

UNIVERSITY OF TORONTO PRESS

© University of Toronto Press, 1967

Reprinted 2017

ISBN 978-0-8020-2043-7 (paper)

P R E F A C E

The present manual is the outgrowth of a series
of lectures on the bacteriology of air given to various
groups of technical and non-technical personnel in many
industrial and research establishments connected with
the supply, moving, and usage of bacteriologically clean
air. These informal sessions were designed to introduce
to "white-room" personnel the idea of bacteriologically
contaminated air and the subsequent air cleaning pro-
cesses. It was found that personnel involved in air
contamination control were generally not exposed to
bacteriology, yet in their daily professional problems
they must often deal with bacteriological monitors,
problems of bacteriological contamination control of
air, and even the manufacture and service of microbial
filtering devices.

Since bacteria and other microorganisms are of
minute dimensions, the problem used to be approached
from the physical point of view of small non-viable
particles in the colloid range. And although many of
the physical properties of small particles of the size
of bacteria are familiar to air contamination personnel,
the property of life added to these microscopic particles adds a factor of complexity and demands a different
approach to the problem, one that has not always been
considered in this modern discipline.

This manual therefore approaches the subject with
elementary concepts of bacteriology and enlarges the
scope of information to the point where it becomes
practically useful and gives the reader a workable understanding of the problems involved in the bacteriological control of air contamination.

The manual is divided into three chapters. Beginning with BASIC PRINCIPLES OF BACTERIOLOGY elementary
ideas pertaining to the problem are presented in a non -
technical manner. The second chapter considers BACTERIO-
LOGY OF AIR and is primarily based on the knowledge and
information presented in the preceding chapter. The last
chapter conveniently unifies the ideas by a practical
approach to THE SAMPLING OF AIRBORNE MICROORGANISMS.

Obviously, it is possible only to scratch the
surface of the problem involved in such an elementary
presentation. But it is hoped that this manual will
provide not only the foundation for further study, but
mainly a workable understanding of the subject, without a stilted and academic approach.

I would like to thank all who helped in any way. Much moral support came from my wife Christine, who was responsible for launching this project. Dr. P. H. Jones, Department of Civil Engineering, University of Toronto, read the original draft of the manuscript. Many of his helpful hints are incorporated in this manual. The editors of the University of Toronto Press, in particular Miss L. Ourom, offered many valuable suggestions. This help is much appreciated.

V. V. K.

October 1967
University of Toronto
Toronto, Canada

C O N T E N T S

BACTERIOLOGY PRIMER IN AIR CONTAMINATION CONTROL

CHAPTER I

B A S I C   P R I N C I P L E S   O F

B A C T E R I O L O G Y

Since time immemorial, man has been classifying things
around him, and so living things came to be designated
as either plant or animal.   However, as scientific
methods were improved,   newer forms of life were dis-
covered which have attributes of both the plant and
animal kingdoms, or which do not fit either of these
categories.   Thus the group Protista was created, to
accommodate all categories of unicellular organisms
that are of microscopic dimensions. The bacteria, being
invisible to the naked eye, unicellular, and not simply
classified as either plant or animal on the basis of
their characteristics, belong to this category.

DISTRIBUTION   OF   BACTERIA

    Bacteria are ubiquitous on earth, but the number
and kinds found vary from place to place, depending on
environmental conditions.   Certain groups of bacteria
can always be identified with particular environments,
the soil harbouring some types of bacteria, while milk,
water, food, the human body, and so on have their own
specific groups of bacteria.   This specificity arises,
because each of these environments can supply certain
types of nutrients, some bacteria being able to metabolize these and thrive while others cannot and perish.
By means of this environmental specificity, bacteria
fall into certain natural groupings.
    Bacteria are also found in air, but one cannot
classify these bacteria as strictly "air bacteria",
as one can the "water bacteria", "milk bacteria", and
so on, because air cannot supply the nutrients needed
for the growth of these organisms. In other words,
there is no such thing as an "air bacterium".   All
bacteria found in air are contaminants, i.e. they have
been introduced into the air by chance or intent, be it
by air currents, smoke, sneezing, coughing, laughing,
speaking, or any other such activity. Nevertheless,
there is hardly a place on earth where bacteria will
not be found in air. Even the air over the oceans, miles
away from any continent or island, shows the presence
of bacteria. The number of bacteria in marine and alpine

air is, however, significantly smaller than in other regions. This is thought to be due to three main reasons: (1) the lack of nutrients in the air, (2) the lack of contaminating factors, and (3) the germicidal effect of ultra-violet light.

Thus the air, although it is not a bacterial habitat, does contain a number of bacteria, the amount of these depending on the activity associated with the environment (Fig. 1) . The air in undisturbed spaces,

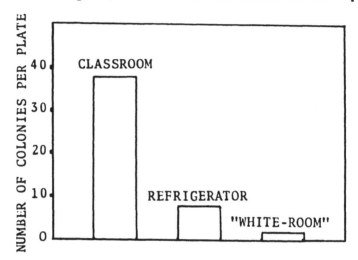

Fig. 1. An example of the relative number of bacteria and fungi from various places grown on a nutrient plate after exposure to the atmosphere for 30 minutes. Incubation time was 48 hours at 34° C.

such as refrigerators, closed rooms, and dust-free areas, in which the air currents are kept at a minimum, will be relatively free from bacteria, because they tend to settle out, while the air in a theatre, a bus, or a gymnasium will contain a large number of bacteria because of the activity associated with such places.

SIZE   AND   SHAPE   OF   BACTERIAL   CELLS

Bacteria are minute organisms. Some measure as much as 80 microns (1 micron = 1 μ = 1/1000 mm or approximately 1/25,000 of an inch) in length, and others as little as 0.2 micron or less. On the average, however, the more common bacteria, including disease - causing ones (which are called *pathogens*), are about 0.5 micron in diameter and 2 to 3 microns in length.

According to shape, bacteria are classified into three main groups (Fig. 2) : rod-shaped bacteria, which are called *bacilli* (sing. *bacillus*); spherical bacteria, called *cocci* (sing. *coccus*); and curved or spiral types of bacteria, called *spirilla* (sing. *spirillum*). All

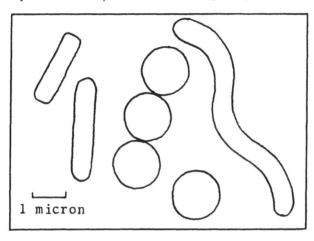

1 micron

Fig. 2. The three common types of bacteria. From the left, the rodlike *bacillus*, the spherical *coccus*, and a spiral form termed *spirillum*.

three types are known to contain pathogenic species, and one cannot definitely say by just looking at a bacterium through a microscope whether or not it is capable of producing disease. Indeed, a multitude of cultural, physical, biochemical, serological, and pathogenicity tests must be performed before an unknown bacterium can be classified. Nevertheless, in hospitals, food and dairy plants, pharmaceutical establishments, public health centres, infectious disease laboratories, and in many "white rooms", where a bacterial contamination may be a hazard, classification of the bacteria found is an important task.

MOTILITY IN BACTERIA

Many bacteria can move from place to place in a fluid or semi - fluid environment. Some bacteria glide over the surface on a layer of slime, while others move rapidly by the action of whiplike projections called *flagella* (sing. *flagellum*), which are very thin, protein

structures, smaller in diameter than the resolution of
the light microscope and therefore not readily observed
unless the flagella are specially treated (Fig. 3).

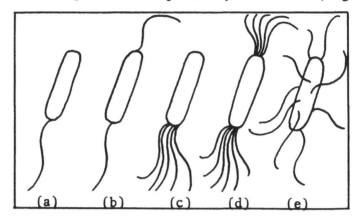

Fig. 3. Main types of bacterial flagellation.
Flagella can be single (a, b) or multiple in a
tuft (c, d), or they can be distributed random-
ly over the whole bacterial surface (e). They
can also arise from one (a, c) or both (b, d)
ends of the organism.

Indirect evidence of the presence of these flagella may
be obtained, however, by the observation of the movement of bacteria in a fluid medium. The spread of
bacteria that are motile in a fluid environment is much
faster than of those bacteria that do not possess flagella or those that cannot glide; but in a dry environment, the spread and establishment of flagellated bacterial organisms is discouraged or kept at a minimum
level. It should be noted that many pathogenic organisms have flagella, but since many non - pathogenic
ones also possess them, the presence of these structures
in itself does not signify that a bacterium is pathogenic.

BACTERIAL   SPORES

Another structure of importance is the bacterial
spore, which is a thick, resistant armour, formed by
some bacteria during periods of unfavourable conditions,
which aids in their survival (Fig. 4). Bacterial spore
formation is not an instantaneous process. In fact, it
is fairly slow and depends on many factors, one of which
is a prerequisite nutrient abundance followed by

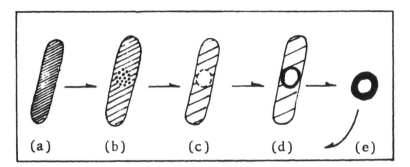

Fig. 4. Diagram of spore formation in a bacterium.
Some bacterial cells can form spores (see text).
This diagram illustrates the progressive changes
from a vegetative form (a) to the spore (e). The
sequence is best thought of as a continuous circle
with stage (e) (the complete spore) later changing
to stage (a) (in a process called germination), if
environmental conditions are optimal for this outgrowth.

unfavourable conditions. Thus, a bacterium that is able
to form a spore (an ability that is determined genetically) must have optimum conditions for growth before
spore formation can proceed. This process is called
sporulation and is in a way a defence mechanism, aiding
the bacterium in survival, because the bacterial spore
can withstand extremely unfavourable conditions, such
as those brought about by heat, cold, disinfection,
desiccation, or radiation. The bacterium must be inside
the spore in order to survive the onslaught of a disinfectant or some other germicidal agent, and cannot
"slip" into its spore when the germicide begins to act.
When the effect of the germicide has worn off, and the
sporulated microbe is again exposed to favourable conditions and optimum temperature, the spore will break
open or slowly dissolve from within, and the bacterium
will emerge (a process called *germination* or *outgrowth*) and begin to grow and to reproduce.

GROWTH   AND   REPRODUCTION   IN   BACTERIA

A bacterium reproduces simply by splitting in two
after it has attained a certain size. This process of
reproduction can be extremely rapid if conditions are
optimal. Thus, for example, a bacterium can produce
another after 20 minutes, and each of the two can give

rise to another after 20 minutes, so that after 40
minutes four bacteria will be present in place of one.
As long as optimum conditions persist the number of
bacteria could continue to double in this way every 20
minutes. Thus, if each of the cells produced continues
to reproduce at the same rate as the original cell, the
number of cells will increase with time in a geometric
progression and can hence be expressed exponentially as
a function of time (Fig. 5).

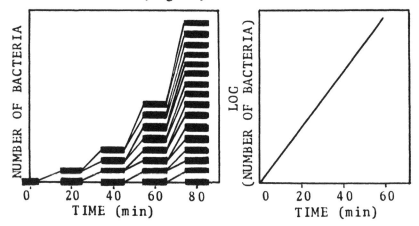

Fig. 5. The left diagram illustrates how one
bacterium (here represented by a short, horizontal bar) multiplies in geometric progression.
The process can be represented in the form of a
straight line when a logarithmic scale is used
(as in diagram on right).

Although under normal circumstances exponential
growth takes place for only a short period of time,
ideally, if a bacterium were to go unchecked in its reproduction for only 24 hours, a single bacterial cell
splitting every 20 minutes would give rise to a progeny
of 2^{72} = 4,722,366,482,869,645,213,696 cells. Assuming
that each cell is 1 micron long and the cells are placed
end to end to form a chain, the chain would reach a
length of approximately 3,000,000,000,000 miles, which
would be sufficient to encircle the earth approximately
120,000,000 times. Fortunately, only very few bacteria
can grow at a rate of one generation every 20 minutes,
and even these must have absolutely perfect nutritional
and environmental conditions to do so.
Thus bacteria are very prolific organisms if optimal conditions for their growth and multiplication can
be maintained for long periods of time. Luckily, this

is not easily possible. In reality, bacteria reproduce for a short period of time until either the food supply becomes depleted or the accumulation of poisonous metabolic by-products becomes growth-limiting, and usually both factors operate simultaneously.

RESULTS   OF   MICROBIAL   GROWTH

As mentioned above, bacteria will grow for only a short time at a rapid rate. After the concentration of nutrients becomes low or the waste products become poisonous through their accumulation, the reproduction rate of a bacterium slows down considerably, with the result that instead of astronomically large numbers of bacteria, we only get small, discrete, confined, and often well manageable areas of bacterial growth. Such localized masses of cells are called *colonies* and unlike individual bacteria, can be easily seen without the aid of a microscope. These colonies are as characteristic as the bacteria that form them and thus aid in the identification of the organisms.

Whenever and wherever bacteria and other microorganisms grow, they bring about a change in their immediate environment. This change is usually manifested as some form of decomposition, sometimes of desirable but usually of undesirable nature, either plainly unpleasant (e.g. the souring of milk) on the one hand, or highly dangerous (e.g. food poisoning) on the other. In air contamination control, however, these effects are only of secondary importance. Of prime importance is, for example, the fact that bacteria, through their terrific rate of multiplication, can and do block some filters, get into air ducts, survive and even multiply in most unsuitable surroundings, thus creating immense contamination problems.

These problems have been recognized for a long time, and although new filters, potent germicides, and sophisticated aerosol sampling devices are continually flooding the market, the terrific potential of bacterial growth does not seem to be realized and is many times simply forgotten. Although this is an observed fact that living things generally resemble their progenitors, there are occasions when this is not necessarily so, when a mutation brings about a sudden change in the hereditary apparatus of the cell. Bacterial mutations occur at a rate of 1 to 1000 for each 10^9 bacteria per generation, but mutation rates can be increased by ultra-violet or X radiation or by the presence of certain chemicals. In terms of air contamination problems this could be illustrated by a hypothetical example. Suppose a bacterial organism has been trapped on a roughing filter of cotton batting. Assume further that some "dirt" has already accumulated on the filter. This dirt may be "food" to the bacterium and the organism will begin to grow and reproduce. Eventually a mass of organisms will be formed, containing over one billion cells. This colony will have from 1 to 1000 or more genetically different cells that differ in some respect from their progenitors. Such mutant bacteria may grow faster than the original type, or they may be more resistant to ultra-violet rays. This means that such mutants may have a better chance of survival in an un-suitable environment, such as presented here by the filter exposed to lethal ultra-violet rays. The rele-vant point here is the fact that although unsuitable growth conditions are present for one type of bacterium, a mutant type may thrive on such changes in the environ-ment. This hypothetical bacterium eventually may clog the filter, or the bacterium will create holes in the filter, and air, dust, bacteria, and other contaminants will find entry into "contamination-free" areas for which the filter was installed, leading to massive con-tamination. Fortunately, most bacterial mutations are *regressive*, but the problem remains, because out of let us say 1000 mutants, there may be one mutant that will exhibit *progressive* characteristics.

Thus a large population of bacterial organisms has the potential of a high degree of variability which is independent of the environmental conditions.

MICROBIAL   NUTRITION

Before a microorganism can grow it must be exposed to two basic types of substances which are classified as nutrients: (1) it must have access to structural units that make up the bacterium and (2) it must have a source of energy for putting these units together, incorporating them into what is called a bacterium, and later must have sufficient energy for the process of division. It must be realized that to be of any use to the bacterium a nutrient must of necessity be of such composition that the bacterial cell can use it as a whole or in part. Even the breaking down of such nutrients into smaller parts requires energy. A sub-stance that is a nutrient to one bacterium is not necessarily a nutrient to another; just as man cannot metabolize cellulose as principal substance so a bac-terium cannot feed on certain types of nutrients.

However, the presence of suitable nutrients per se does
not necessarily result in bacterial growth. Factors
like temperature, pH, moisture, presence or absence of
oxygen, to name but a few, play an important part in
microbial nutrition. Some of the more important factors
affecting the growth of bacteria are mentioned in the
following section.

It can be safely stated that as a group bacteria
are omnivorous and that they can live, grow, and multiply in the most extreme and the most unlikely milieu
that this earth has to offer, be it in natural surroundings or in synthetic environments. In fact, the
most remarkable metabolic feat of bacteria is their
utilization of modern organic compounds that have never
occurred in the history of the earth and can be found
only in the synthetic chemist's laboratory. This adapt-
ability goes so far, to mention another example, that
bacteria not only utilize, but in some cases have grown
to be dependent on some potent protoplasmic poisons
(e.g. cyanide, carbon monoxide, some antibiotics) as
food sources.

Basically, bacteria can be divided into two categories, depending on whether or not they can synthesize
essential food-stuff and thus are or are not self -
sufficient. In other words, there are bacteria that can
only utilize already preformed (organic) substances
and there are others that can make these from simple,
elementary (inorganic) substances. No matter to what
group a bacterium belongs, one principle is clear:
a bacterial cell must obtain food and must obtain the
energy to live, to grow, and to reproduce in order to
survive. This can happen in the presence of atmospheric
oxygen or in its absence, since some bacteria do not
require molecular oxygen to survive, and in fact may
become inactivated in the presence of air. The complete
removal of molecular oxygen from an environment may
only enhance the growth of some microbes. However,
whether or not oxygen is available, nutrients must be
at hand before growth can occur.

SURFACE   PROPERTIES   OF   BACTERIAL   CELLS

The living matter that makes up bacterial cells
is confined to the bacterium by a thick external barrier
called the *cell wall*, consisting of several thick and
thin layers, each having a definite function of its own,
but interrelated with the others so as to make a whole.
This orderly conglomeration of coats and membranes is
by no means a passive element, but has living and dynamic

properties which influence the environment of the bacterium, but the surface of the bacterial cell is influenced by the environment also and at times it is difficult to distinguish the cause from the effect.

Many of the surface properties of bacteria can be understood in terms of physicochemical concepts developed for the non-biological sciences, but only the electric charge will be discussed here, as it is concerned directly in many problems of air contamination control associated with the electrostatic precipitation of small particles.

The fact that bacteria exhibit an electric charge is observed when bacteria move in an electric field in particular directions. Under normal conditions of growth and when pH values are around neutrality, bacteria tend to migrate to the anode, indicating that their surfaces are negatively charged. This property is now universally employed in electrostatic precipitation of bacteria from air streams passing over plates that are positively charged. However, for many bacteria the surface charge changes during the growth cycle of the organism; thus a young organism exhibits a drop in electrophoretic mobility, but this rises after the bacterial cell gets older. Furthermore, the pH of the medium (such as in an aerosol particle in which a bacterium may be trapped) tends to influence the surface charge of a bacterial cell. For this reason, although bacteria can be safely said to carry a negative charge at neutral pH, when the hydrogen ion concentration reaches fairly acidic values the charge of the bacterial surface becomes positive. Some bacteria also seem to reverse to a positive charge when subjected to pH values of 13.0 or higher. From the above it can be seen that when the surface chemistry is varied, the surface charge of bacteria is varied also. These matters are even more complicated when bacteria occur in clumps, or when pathogenic bacteria are considered, since they usually possess an extra envelope (termed a *capsule*) which has specific determinant groups that affect the final ionic distribution and thus the electric charge on the surface. It is unimportant to consider the charges in the interior of the cell, as these do not affect the electrophoretic migration of the cell, but factors such as temperature, viscosity of the medium, and the net strength of the field definitely influence the rate of migration of bacterial cells in an electric field.

It is suggested that, in the light of these facts, manufacturers of electrostatic precipitating devices instal a negatively charged plate to minimize the non - precipitation of positively charged bacterial organisms and hence make their devices more efficient.

12

EFFECTS OF PHYSICAL AND CHEMICAL AGENTS ON
BACTERIA

The effect of various physical and chemical agents
on bacteria in general has been known for a long time.
Heat, light, pressure, desiccation, vibration, and electric current are only some of the examples of physical
agents. In addition, an immense number of chemicals
are known to affect bacteria; among these the more common and better known are alcohol, antibiotics, arsenics,
dyes, and quinine. It is important to stress the point
that bacterial spores are affected to a much less degree when exposed to an unfavourable environment (be it
physical or chemical in nature) than are actively growing (*vegetative*) bacterial cells.

Heat influences the growth of bacteria in three
different ways:

1. All bacteria can live in a range of temperatures,
but only at one particular temperature will the microbes
thrive better than at other temperatures. This is the
optimum temperature for their growth.

2. Bacteria can withstand high (*maximum*) and low
(*minimum*) temperatures, but their growth is impaired
at the two extremes. Bacteria resist low temperatures
better than high temperatures.

3. When the temperature of the environment in which
the microbe lives passes beyond the maximum temperature,
the bacterium will be killed. This principle is utilized
in the process of heat sterilization (this is an absolute destruction of all living matter), which is most
effective when it is done in the presence of moisture.
Desiccation, or the removal of water, also causes the
death of bacteria, as moisture is essential to living
organisms.

Sunlight is known to have a killing effect on
bacteria and moulds, killing action being attributed to
a component of sunlight--ultra-violet rays. Ultra-violet lights are produced commercially and are in use in
hospitals and sterile rooms, where they aid in keeping
the bacterial population at a minimum. However, ultra -
violet germicidal lamps are useless in dirty and dusty
areas, because the power of penetration of ultra-violet
radiation is limited. Bacteria under a layer of dirt
are not affected by ultra-violet radiation, because the
radiation becomes absorbed by the dust particles cover-
ing the bacteria.

With regard to chemical agents, it must be empha-
sized that not all chemical agents have a deleterious
effect on bacteria, and that some chemicals are more

13

effective at lower concentrations than at a higher one. Alcohol, for example, is more germicidal at a concentration of 70 per cent than at 95 per cent or higher. Any chemical agent that *kills* bacteria or other microorganisms is termed a *disinfectant* (or *germicide*). Any chemical substance that *stops*, *inhibits*, or *prevents* the growth of bacteria without necessarily killing them is called a *bacteriostatic* agent.

Addendum: A WORD ON MOULDS, YEASTS, AND VIRUSES

Although bacteriology deals specifically with bacteria, there are a variety of other small organisms with which a bacteriologist always comes in contact. These minute organisms are moulds (fungi), yeasts, and viruses. They have many similar properties, and are, therefore, conveniently grouped in one common science, namely *microbiology*. Many properties that have been discussed above in connection with bacteria apply also to these three groups of organisms, although it must be stated emphatically that categorical differences exist between the above groups, and that whatever applies to one does not necessarily apply to another. For better understanding of the differences involved, the interested reader should refer to some of the treatises on microbiology mentioned at the end of this chapter.

CONCLUSION

The foregoing basic principles of bacteriology have been written in as simple a manner as possible, so that many details have had to be omitted. The author is not aware of any publication that deals specifically with bacteriology from the point of view of air contamination control, although the works cited at the end of this chapter have good discussions on many aspects of the subject with which a modern air contamination control technician should be familar. Readers who are interested in pursuing this subject in more detail and with greater emphasis on specific points are referred to these volumes.

GLOSSARY

NOTE: This short glossary contains all important technical terms in this chapter. Some terms not encountered are also included, because they are often popularly misinterpreted.

AGAR: A gelatinlike substance obtained from certain seaweed, which is non-nutritive to most bacteria. When dissolved in boiling water and cooled, it sets to a firm jelly, which is used as a base for growing bacteria.

ANTIBIOTIC: A growth-inhibiting substance produced by microorganisms.

ANTISEPTIC: A substance that prevents or inhibits the growth of microorganisms without necessarily destroying them.

AUTOCLAVE: An apparatus for sterilizing by steam under pressure.

BACILLUS (plural, BACILLI): A rod-shaped bacterium.

BACTERIOLOGY: The science that deals with bacteria.

BACTERIUM (plural, BACTERIA): A microscopic, one-celled organism, not necessarily pathogenic.

COCCUS (plural, COCCI): A bacterium that is round (spherical) in shape.

COLONY: A distinct, isolated group of bacteria growing in a nutrient environment and visible to the naked eye.

CULTURE: A general growth of microorganisms.

DISINFECTANT: A (chemical) agent that kills microbes; also called a germicide.

DROPLET INFECTION: Infection by means of small droplets thrown into the air while talking, coughing, or sneezing, and usually harbouring pathogenic microorganisms which may remain alive for hours.

FLAGELLUM (plural, FLAGELLA): A whiplike structure in microorganisms used for motility.

GERM: A general term usually referring to a pathogenic bacterium, but also used popularly in connection with viruses.

GERMICIDE: See DISINFECTANT.

GERMINATION: A state of sudden active growth after an inactive period; usually associated with a spore.

GROWTH MEDIUM: See NUTRIENT MEDIUM.

INFECTION: Invasion of body tissues by pathogenic organisms which multiply and cause disease.

LIQUID MEDIUM: A liquid nutrient medium for growing microorganisms.

MEDIUM: Any suitable growth environment for microorganisms.

MICROBE: Germ.

MICRON: A unit of measurement (written as μ) representing 1/1000 of a millimeter or approximately 1/25,000 of an inch.

MIXED CULTURE: A growth of two or more types of microorganisms in the same nutrient medium.

MOULD: Usually a multicellular, plantlike organism of microscopic dimensions, lacking chlorophyll.

MULTICELLULAR: Consisting of many cells.

NON-PATHOGENIC: Not producing or causing disease.

NUTRIENT MEDIUM: A medium containing the necessary food-stuff for microorganisms.

PATHOGENIC: Causing or producing disease.

PURE CULTURE: A growth of only one type of microorganism in a medium.

SOLID MEDIUM: A medium containing gelatin or agar.

SPIRILLUM (plural, SPIRILLA): A spiral-shaped bacterium.

SPORE: A partially inactive state in some bacteria, characterized by the presence of a tough protective coat resistant to many chemical, physical, and biological agents.

STERILIZATION: The process of freeing completely from all living matter.

UNICELLULAR: Consisting of a single cell.

ULTRA-VIOLET RAYS: Rays of certain wavelengths having germicidal properties.

VEGETATIVE CELL (as contrasted to *SPORE*): An actively growing cell.

VIRULENT: Able to produce disease.

BIBLIOGRAPHY

P. L. Carpenter (1967), Microbiology (2nd ed.; Philadelphia: W. B. Saunders Co.).

M. J. Pelczar, Jr. and R. D. Reid (1965), Microbiology (2nd ed.; New York: McGraw-Hill Book Co., Inc.).

A. J. Salle (1967), Fundamental Principles of Bacteriology (6th. ed.; New York: McGraw-Hill Book Co., Inc.).

R. Y. Stanier, M. Doudoroff, and E. A. Adelberg (1963), The Microbial World (2nd. ed.; Englewood Cliffs, N. J.: Prentice-Hall).

W. W. Umbreit (1962), Modern Microbiology (San Francisco: W. H. Freeman and Co.).

G. S. Wilson and A. A. Miles (1964), Topley and Wilson's Principles of Bacteriology and Immunity (5th ed.; London: Edward Arnold, Ltd.).

CHAPTER II

B A C T E R I O L O G Y   O F   A I R

Air contains not only a mixture of gases (approximately
78% nitrogen, 21% oxygen, and mixtures of argon, carbon
dioxide, and hydrogen) and water vapour, but also various microscopic and submicroscopic particles referred
to as particulate contamination. The term "contaminant"
usually includes pollen, dust, bacteria, yeasts, moulds,
etc., which are present in various amounts, depending
on the location of the sample taken. As has been mentioned in Chapter I, air does not provide the essential
food-stuff for the growth and reproduction of bacteria,
or for any other type of microorganism, and as such
cannot be considered a habitat suited for microbes. It
is best to think of microorganisms in the air as trav-
ellers that have not yet reached their destination.
Such a concept is useful not only from the medical point
of view, but also from the point of view of contamination control, as will be seen later.

The density of animal and human populations in the
area, the amount of vegetation, the temperature, the
humidity, air currents, the extent and nature of the
soil all contribute to the amount of the bacteria found
in the air as well as to the quality of the collected
sample, and hazards -- medical and non-medical. Whereas
public health authorities are concerned with air contaminants that present a medical hazard and may not
bother much with other contaminants, air contamination
personnel must be familiar with all types. The fact
that contamination of whatever sort is present where it
should not be should be the chief concern. As long as
this problem is tackled successfully, contamination of
infectious and non-infectious nature can be checked.

Although microorganisms will be the principal ob-
jects of discussion in this chapter it should be kept
in mind that non-living contaminants should be treated
similarly, and with no less respect. This point can be
illustrated by an example taken from a pharmaceutical
manufacturer producing sterile products (those products
destined for injection). The control department will
necessarily reject any lot of ampoules that show the
presence of particulate matter, like lint or dust,
when tested, whether there be bacterial growth or not.

18

DEFINITIONS OF CONCEPTS

Airborne microorganisms can occur in three different forms, or rather in three different environmental associations, which can be broadly classified as follows: (1) dust particles, (2) droplets, and (3) droplet nuclei. It may be of value to define these concepts to minimize confusion.

Dust particles are generally relatively large pieces of dried material, and may be of animal, vegetable, or mineral origin. They are easily stirred up by air currents and may or may not remain suspended in the air. They may be said to represent the principal form of particulate contamination and also the most frequent one. This form of contamination is easier to control than the other two forms. Since bacteria and other microorganisms found in the air are rarely free but are usually found attached to dust particles, they are thus easily immobilized if means are developed for trapping the dust particles. It should be noted that bacteria associated with dust contamination in outside air rarely have pathogenic significance, being considered *saprobes* (organisms that live on dead organic matter). However, the conditions of air indoors are quite different and such a rule cannot be applied.

A very important aspect to consider in dust contamination is the fact that bacteria and moulds can form spores (see Chapter I) and thus can resist unfavourable conditions for long periods of time. The definition of dust given above is not very precise, but is made in that way on purpose. Thus, for instance, secretions that leave the mouth in a moist form cannot be spoken of as dust. On the other hand, if such secretions get into clothing and soak in and leave a dry crust of particulate matter, they do form dust particles which can easily contaminate the air. It is important to keep in mind the various ways in which dust can arise, directly or indirectly.

Particulate contamination (and this includes microorganisms) can also be associated with droplets, which can be of biological or of physicochemical origin. A sneeze, for example, is of biological origin and will most probably contain a large number of microbes. Droplets of biological origin are formed and expelled into the air during whistling, laughing, coughing, speaking, washing, pipetting, and a legion of other activities associated with everyday life. Droplets of physicochemical origin may arise from any activity entailing

the dispensing of liquids or semi-liquids not containing living matter. Thus, one "white room" known to the
author contained a water fountain to which white-room
personnel had continued access, and this created a contamination hazard. During the process of turning on a
water tap various-sized droplets are formed. The fate
of these ejected droplets depends on their size, on the
force of their ejection from the tap, and the environment. A droplet 1 mm in diameter may be projected a fair
distance and fall to the ground soon after, while smaller droplets (less than 0.1 mm in diameter) will be carried away by air currents and will evaporate rapidly,
leaving a residue termed droplet nuclei. Early investi-
gators (Flügge, 1897; Winslow and Robinson, 1910) came
to the conclusion that the number of small droplets of
respiratory origin that remain suspended in the air is
so small that they can be regarded as negligible in
causing infections. Other workers (notably Wells and
Wells, 1936), however, have pointed out the infectious
hazards associated with such droplet nuclei, by demon-
strating their longevity and their wide distribution by
air currents as well. It was Jennison (1942) who showed
that more than 20,000 tiny droplets are formed during a
sneeze, and that the smaller their diameter, the faster
they evaporate, forming droplet nuclei in air and become
dispersed (see Fig. 6).

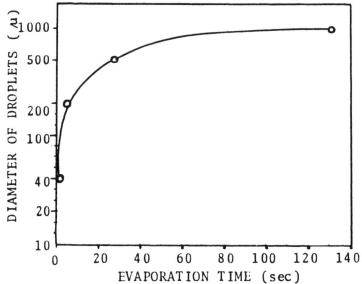

Fig. 6. Relation between diameter of water
droplets and their evaporation time in un-
saturated, still air at 22° C (curve plotted
from data of Jennison, 1942).

The residue of droplet nuclei formed by the evaporation of droplets is fine enough to be carried by the smallest air current, but if droplet nuclei are formed in still air, they settle out according to the well-known law of Stokes, which defines the velocity (v) of a small sphere falling under the action of gravity (g) through a viscous medium (here air) as being constant, depending on the radius of the sphere (r), the density of the sphere (d), the coefficient of viscosity of the medium (K), and the density of the medium (D):

$$v = \frac{2gr^2 (d - D)}{9K} \quad .$$

About 1×10^4 to 1×10^6 droplet nuclei can be formed from a single sneeze, of which about 50 per cent contain microorganisms (Duguid, 1946). However, the pathogenic organisms seem to be associated with only the larger particles, namely those of diameter 4 to 20 microns (Noble, Lidwell, and Kingston, 1963).

CONTROL   OF   AIRBORNE   MICROORGANISMS

The epidemiology of airborne infections will not be considered here. It should be mentioned, however, that many microbiological pathogens can remain viable in droplets for days, and that the droplet nucleus is the primary mode of spread for many diseases when there is close association between people such as may exist in theatres, army barracks, hospital wards, or vehicles of public transportation. Microbiological droplet formation can usually be effectively controlled by simple principles of personal hygiene, but the control of dust and of droplet nuclei depends on the effective use of controlled ventilation coupled with disinfectant vapours, dust suppressors, air filters, and ultra-violet irradiation. It is known that a damp and humid atmosphere contains fewer microorganisms than does dry air under similar conditions. This is explained by the fact that humid air is actually a collection of droplets of moisture which slowly settle and in the process carry off and trap microorganisms. Thus in late fall, winter, and early spring the number of microorganisms in the air is much smaller than in the dry summer season (see Fig. 7). But there are also daily variations in the airborne microorganism count, and counts of airborne cells of bacteria or fungi in one area differ from those

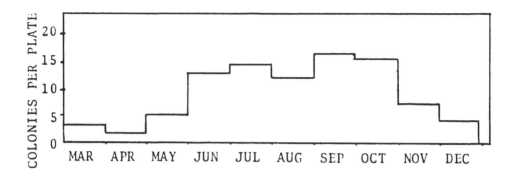

Fig. 7. Monthly average of colonies per plate
per 30 minutes exposure in suburban Toronto,1963.
Medium was nutrient agar. Incubation was 48 hours
at 34° C. Colonies were bacterial and fungal.

in another area, depending on geographical location,
prevailing winds, season, time of day, and, of course,
the method of collection of the sample, including the
type of medium employed and the temperature of incubation. From this point of view it is not only impracti-
cal but also quite impossible to set or even suggest
control limits for airborne microbial contamination.
This goes only for outside air. Each investigator must
determine an average count of airborne contamination
for his own specific area or location using a method
that is best suited for his purposes (see Chapter III)
and not consider absolute values but recognize *trends*.
     The control of airborne microorganisms indoors
is a different problem. Continuous disinfection of in-
door air (or air destined for indoors) can be accomplished by: (1) destruction of microorganisms by ultra-
violet irradiation; (2) collection of particles by
electrostatic precipitation; (3) trapping of microorganisms through the use of fluids; (4) suppression
or elimination of dust.

Destruction of Microorganisms by Ultra-violet Irradiation

     The most potent and most effective ultra-violet
rays for the destruction of microorganisms are those of
wavelength approximately 2600 Å . These are destructive
to microorganisms because they affect and destroy the
most vital of all microbial sub-structures necessary
for reproduction, namely, deoxyribonucleic acid (DNA).

However, the effect of ultra-violet light on the steri-
lity of air is closely dependent on the humidity of
the air, the state of suspension of the particles, the
total exposure time, the force of air currents, the
strength of the ray, and so on. There are thus many var-
iants to consider, although some of these may be controlled by the use of certain devices before actual irradiation, such as a series of filters or dehumidifiers.

Collection of Particles by Electrostatic Precipitation

Most microorganisms can be collected by electrostatic precipitation, because they usually exhibit polarity in an electric field (see Chapter I). Hence,
the device for electrostatic precipitation is usually
put first in the chain of devices employed for the pu-
rification of air. Problems may arise, however, in
highly contaminated conditions, when clumps of organisms
or particles occur which may not exhibit any polarity
at all, and consequently may not be precipitated, but
their collection may be achieved by other devices later
in the chain.

Trapping of Microorganisms in Fluids

Under the term fluids are grouped all vapours,
mists, or fluid controls, which are sometimes also referred to as "air washing" or "air scrubbing" devices
and having germistatic or germicidal properties. For
smaller rooms sprays of hypochlorous acid (Edward and
Lidwell, 1943) are efficient for the control of airborne
organisms, but the effectiveness of such aerosols depends
on the amount of moisture present in the air (Elford and
van den Ende, 1945), the compound being most germicidal
in a concentration of 0.1 to 0.3 ppm with relative
humidity between 70 and 90 per cent.
The more modern method is to employ a device that
impinges any microorganism present in the air being
treated into a germicidal or germistatic solution with
a high surface tension, which traps the organisms.

Suppression or Elimination of Dust

Suppression of dust is the easiest method of air
sanitation and has been successfully employed in various institutions by the controlled oiling of floors and
textiles. The controlling action is strictly mechanical,
but is quite effective in places such as hospital wards
or army barracks.
The elimination of dust particles is best achieved

by filtration of incoming air. There are problems inherent in this operation, such as the clogging of filters, seen especially if the pore size is too small and the contamination rate is too high, or ineffectiveness when the filter pores are too large and some of the trapped microorganisms may work their way through the filter. In the latter case, the arrival of the microorganisms or the particles in the area being treated is simply delayed and the contamination is not eliminated. The effectiveness of filters in eliminating dust particles or microorganisms is therefore limited, and when they are used, it is necessary to inspect and replace them at frequent intervals.

It is important to realize that not one of these methods is 100 per cent effective by itself, but if two or more of these methods are used in series, the retention of particles increases enormously and significantly. Generally, the electrostatic precipitator is put first, then the filtration unit, followed by the air scrubbing device and exposure to ultra-violet light, and optionally an ultra-filtration unit is added at the end of the treatment (see Fig. 8).

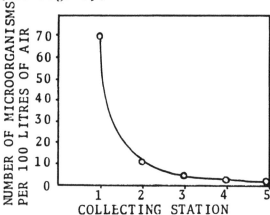

Fig. 8. Effects of reduction of airborne microorganisms by the use of series of decontamination devices. Sampling was done by capillary impinger into saline. Culturing was accomplished by transfer to nutrient agar and 48-hour incubation at 34° C. Collecting station: 1, before electrostatic precipitation; 2, after electrostatic precipitation and filter; 3, after air scrubbing unit; 4, after ultra-violet irradiation; 5, after ultra-filtration, just before delivery to sterile area. (Data from Kingsley, 1964.)

EFFECTIVENESS OF SAMPLING vs. EFFECTIVENESS OF COLLECTION

There is one very important aspect to be borne in mind, namely, that the collection of microorganisms from the air is only as good as the process of collection itself, even though a sampling device may give a different picture. In other words, let us say 100 organisms are purposely impinged on an air cleaning device, and the device collects only 50 of the original 100 organisms and lets the rest through, and then an aerosol sampler monitors the treated air and finds only 25 organisms in it. This indicates a higher effectiveness of the sanitation device than is actually the case (75% in comparison with 50%). Thus, since air filtration may be many times worse than air sampling may indicate, the problem of determining the efficiency of air sampling devices is one of great importance in air sanitation. This problem will be discussed in Chapter III.

LITERATURE CITED

J. P. Duguid (1946), "The Size and Duration of Air-Carriage of Respiratory Droplets and Droplet Nuclei," _J. Hyg._ 44: 47.

D. G. Edward and O. M. Lidwell (1943), "Studies on Air-borne Virus Infection, III," _J. Hyg. 43:_ 196.

W. J. Elford and J. van den Ende (1945), "Studies on the Disinfecting Action of Hypochlorous Acid Gas and Sprayed Solution of Hypochlorite Against Bacterial Aerosols," _J. Hyg._ 44: 1.

C. Flugge (1897), "Ueber Luftinfektion," _Ztsch. f. Hyg._ 25: 179.

M. W. Jennison (1942), "Atomizing of Mouth and Nose Secretions into the Air as Revealed by High-Speed Photography," in _Aerobiology_ (Publication No. 17 of the AAAS), p. 106.

V. V. Kingsley (1964), "Pharmaceutical Sterile Areas", _Air. Eng._ 6: 28.

W. C. Noble, O. M. Lidwell, and D. Kingston (1963), "The Size Distribution of Air-borne Particles Carrying Micro-organisms," _J. Hyg._ 61: 385.

W. F. Wells and Mildred W. Wells (1936), "Air-borne
    Infection," J.A.M.A. 107: 1698, 1805.

C. E. A. Winslow and E. A. Robinson (1910), "An In-
    vestigation of the Extent of the Bacterial Pollu-
    tion of the Atmosphere by Mouth Spray," J. Inf.
    Dis. 7: 17.

CHAPTER III

THE SAMPLING OF AIRBORNE

MICROORGANISMS

One usually associates bacterial contamination with
hospitals, nurseries, and biological establishments.
However, it is not necessarily restricted to these
areas. Personnel that have to deal with the more sophisticated instrumentation that is continually being
developed, must deal increasingly with biological particles, in addition to non-living contamination, in
whatever area in which they are working. For this reason
they must be familiar with a few techniques of sampling
airborne microorganisms and with the respective merits
of the different sampling methods. It is not the purpose
of this chapter to show how various groups of microorganisms can be identified after collection but to state
the comparative merits of various air sampling devices.
Only general bacterial sampling methods of contaminated
air will be discussed, with no direct mention of manufacturers' products or trade marks, but at the end of
the chapter a number of manufacturers are listed for
the convenience of the interested reader, who might wish
to obtain more information on a particular device by
writing direct to the manufacturer. The choice of manufacturer does not necessarily imply acceptance of his
product by the author, but is intended only as reference.

IMPORTANCE   OF   THE   CRITERION   OF   CONTAMINATION

When an air sampler collects particles from the air,
whether they be of biological or of non-biological nature,
their quantitative evaluation is the weakest link in the
chain, beginning with filtration of the air and termi-
nating with species identification, and hence the limit-
ing factor.

In many institutions the criterion of air contamination may rest on or be expressed as the number of
viable organisms collected in an air sample. In other
establishments the same criterion of viability may still
hold, but the associated size distribution of the collected particles may be an added factor to consider. In
other concerns, not only biological but also particulate
contamination of non-biological nature must be collected,
studied, and evaluated. It is for such reasons as these

that before a study of air contamination is begun, definite, clear-cut criteria must be established for the
limits of control and evaluation. One should keep in
mind, for example, that bacteria can contaminate the air
in more than one manner (see Chapter II), that spores of
microorganisms are present in the air, and that many external factors influence the biological contaminant with
regard to its viability and its spread over long dis-
tances as well (see Chapters I and II). It would be
worthless, for instance, to initiate and complete an
extensive evaluation programme of airborne contamination
with regard to viability of organisms, if the information needed was that of *all* particulate contamination,
whether viable or not. Although one sampler or technique may give the right answers, some other method may
utterly fail in this regard. There are many types of
samplers, and the selection of a particular device for
a specific air-monitoring programme may prove rather
difficult if the information desired is not known be-
forehand, or if the performance limits of the sampler
are unknown.

TYPES   OF   AIR-MONITORING   DEVICES

Fundamentally, there are only two methods by which
one can collect airborne microorganisms: (1) by collection into liquids and (2) by collection onto solids.
Each of these methods has a number of variations, but
the most important criterion must be the preservation
of the viability of the collected organisms. These two
general methods can, of course, be applied to the evaluation of non-biological contamination of air in addition to the biological, and airborne microorganisms may
be collected by trapping them in some liquid that has
no germicidal qualities. When sampling is done by the
collection of organisms from the air on solid surfaces,
then the viability of the organisms gathered depends
strongly on the rapidity of transfer into a suitable
growth medium, as well as on other factors, such as
humidity and temperature. If the various factors that
are involved are closely controlled and taken into con-
sideration when evaluating data, an accurate duplication
can be achieved. However, results obtained by one method
of air sampling can never be taken and compared to a
different method of collecting airborne microorganisms.

Gravitational Settling

One of the oldest and simplest methods of monitoring airborne microorganisms is to expose a number of
sterile plates containing a jellylike nutrient substance

(Koch, 1881). This can be done in either a random or a previously arranged pattern in a room or area and the exposure time can vary from 15 minutes to several hours, depending on the activity and the information desired. The plates are subsequently incubated at a suitable temperature so that developed colonies of microorganisms can be counted with ease. There are two main points to remember when using this method. First, only the larger dust particles and droplets floating in the air will settle out in a reasonable time, because their settling behaviour is governed less by air currents than by forces of gravitation and their direction of movement is vertically downward and not diagonal or horizontal as for droplet nuclei and similar small particles, which do not settle out to any appreciable degree in a turbulent environment and sometimes take many hours to settle in still air. Thus, a sphere 1.0 micron in diameter having a specific gravity of 1.0 will settle in still air (at 70° F) 5.04 inches in an hour, while a sphere 10 microns in diameter under similar conditions will settle at a rate of 6.07 inches every minute, or 364.2 inches in an hour.

The second point to remember is that this method is excellent and very effective when qualitative results are wanted, but is of no use when accurate, immediate, quantitative results are sought. However, in long-term or continuous programmes the information obtained is of use to indicate *trends*.

A slight variation on this method is employed for non-viable counts, in which microscope glass slides (1 x 3 inches), instead of Petri plates with a nutrient medium, are exposed to the air and are then examined under a microscope and conveniently stored for reference (Marsh et al., 1962).

Filtration

Air filtration is very effective in some air - monitoring devices. The filters can be sponge type, or made of fibres, or consist of a porous membrane. The construction and make-up of these is important and play a part in the viability evaluation. Thus, if a sponge-type filter is employed, the material of which it is made must be of such make-up that it can be easily as well as rapidly broken down, freeing entrapped organisms. If this can be achieved to only a small degree or not at all, the evaluation will be wrong.

With filters that are made of fibres a similar breakdown must be accomplished before lodged bacteria can be freed and thus evaluated. For this reason, only those fibre filters in which the fibres are not too

29

compact should be used to keep the resistance to air flow low and to ensure an accurate evaluation of collected viable particles, because complete fibre dispersion must be accomplished when the fibre is shaken in a liquid nutrient medium. It should be noted that with this type of monitor it is not the collected number of bacterial particles but the number of organisms that is evaluated, because the shaking breaks up bacterial clumps into smaller subunits (cells).

Membrane filters do not have to be fragmented before evaluation, because the collected microorganisms tend to stay on the surface, the pores being smaller than the collected organisms. Thus, whereas membrane filters are true screens, the sponge and fibre filter types cannot be so called, because the collected organisms penetrate some distance below the collection surface, the openings being larger than the collected particles and collection being usually achieved by trapping the organisms in small spaces or crevices created by the various niches of the sponge or angles of the fibres. The membrane-type filter has the advantage that one can use membranes of various pore sizes, and can thus simultaneously size the particles and carry out a qualitative and quantitative evalutation.

One important aspect of the membrane-type filters that is rarely mentioned in the literature is the generation of electrostatic forces on the membrane filter surface. Negative charges are set up and held for long periods of time on the filter, preventing passage of far smaller particles than the pore dimensions of the filter may indicate. This may or may not be desirable. In addition, with small pores clogging may become a problem in heavily contaminated conditions, but by using a prefilter some of this clogging may be eliminated.

Deposition by Centrifugation

This method is an ingenious variation on the simple deposition of particles by sedimentation. It utilizes centrifugal force as the depositing power. Airborne particles subjected to this sampling technique are impacted at a higher rate than simple gravitational sedimentation can ever hope to achieve. Consequently, shorter assay periods are required, but the devices (which are not used often now) are not much more efficient or cheaper than some other air monitors. It must be pointed out also that these devices pick up particles that achieve a velocity of approximately 30 feet/hour under normal gravitational settling, which would correspond to a spherical particle of specific gravity 1.0 having a diameter of about 10 microns. The collection of particles that have a lower settling velocity is only 67 per cent effective.

30

Electrostatic Precipitators

Large amounts of air can be sampled by electrostatic precipitation. The principle of the device rests on the observation that many particles are either electrically charged or can be made to be so prior to their attraction to negatively or positively charged plates. The collection proper, however, is made either by impinging or impacting the particles by placing liquid or semi-solid media in the tortuous path of the air being sampled. Since negative *and* positive particles must be collected, there is need for two types of collection plates. This must not be forgotten during the evaluation of the results, because each collecting unit will have only the negatively charged particles or only the positively charged particles. However, the disadvantages, such as the presence of high voltage, which necessitates careful handling; the complexity of the device, which demands constant attention in its setting up and maintenance; the high sampling rate, which may cause desiccation of the sample if glass or other solid surfaces are employed; and, finally, the lack of studies of bacteria subjected to high voltages make this monitoring device not only awkward and undesirable to use, but bacteriologically unacceptable.

Slit Samplers, Drum Samplers, Multijet Monitors, and Solid Surface Impactors

The term "solid surface" is sometimes ambiguous, because it may also denote a "semi-solid surface", such as one of agar or gelatin, as well as a strictly solid surface like glass. To minimize confusion here, "solid surface" will only apply to collection surfaces made of any material other than agar or gelatin.

Slit samplers are one of the most effective types of devices for the enumeration of microorganisms. The earliest sampler made by Bourdillon et al. (1941) was improved in 1946 (Luckiesh, Taylor, and Holloday), and consists of a Petri plate with nutrient agar enclosed in a metal and plastic housing, revolving under a radial slit at a predetermined rate. The air is drawn through the sampler by a vacuum at a rate of approximately 1 cfm, but when it passes through the approximately 0.25 mm wide slit, the air velocity reaches 100 ft/sec, so that positive impaction of airborne particles is effected on the agar. Even the smaller airborne contaminants are collected because the air passage is in close proximity to the impacting surface. The advantage of the revolving device is obvious, because it clearly pin-points the exact time of appearance of contamination, and thus correlates it with incidents taking place in the environment being sampled. Whereas the ability to determine the time factor is the more obvious and important attribute of this type of air sampler, its characteristics and qualities of effectiveness, complete viability, and the metering of air-flow rates should not be underestimated. However, two factors must be kept in mind: (1) it is not the absolute number of particles in the air that is measured, but the number of impacted contaminants (in other words, clumps of organisms are rarely broken up), and (2) only short time periods can be considered.

Drum samplers were introduced by Andersen and Andersen (1961). The air is drawn in and impacted by means of a vacuum from periods ranging from 24 minutes to 24 hours at sampling rates varying from 0.1 to 3.0 litres per minute. A unique design guides the impaction line in a helical path, thus increasing the length of the available surface immensely to approximately 456 inches, as compared to the Petri plate slit sampler, with a path length of about 12 inches. The merits of this sampler are many and it is effective from many points of view.

Multijet monitors are available for collection, enumeration, and differential sizing of airborne contamination in one stage. Thus, Andersen (1958) reports the automatic separation and collection of airborne microorganisms in six different size categories, by employing successively smaller jet pore sizes from 0.0465 inch diameter at the first stage right down to 0.0100 inch diameter in the last stage. The corresponding jet velocities increase by a factor of more than 20. The advantage of this device is the automatic sizing of viable and non-viable particles in the air sample into easily recognizable hazardous and non-hazardous aerodynamic ranges (i.e. sizes that penetrate the lungs and those that do not).

Strictly *solid surface impactors* should not be considered together with bacteriological air monitors, because the impactors deposit the sampled particles on solid surfaces such as glass, plastic, membranes, or paper. Potentially viable particles will have a small chance of surviving and such devices are unreliable with regard to viability studies, but if rapid and appropriate methods for the cultivation of microorganisms are available after the sampling is over, they may give a reasonably quantitative estimate of airborne fungi and bacteria that are carried by the collected

particles. Generally speaking, however, these impactors
are of use only in dust, pollen, and radioactive particle analysis, and do not give the actual particle count,
but densitometer readings of the concentration of the
collected particles on an area of predetermined size
(e.g. 10 mm^2). A piece of paper or a long tape can be
used with these impactors for purposes of continuous
monitoring. As these samplers give relative results, the
author does not feel that they are suitable for the
monitoring of the bacterial contamination of air, no
matter how useful they are for dust sampling, or in air
pollution control.

Liquid (Capillary) Impingers

One of the most effective methods for bacterial
air sampling is to draw a stream of air at high velocity
through or into a liquid. All particles that are in the
air sample thus treated will be brought in contact with
the liquid, wetted, and held there by surface tension.
However, the velocity of the drawn air should not be
made to approach sonic proportions, because the actively growing (vegetative) cells of certain organisms tend
to be disrupted and die. Subsonic sampling is thus recommended; with it the collecting efficiency does not
suffer appreciably and the delicate cells of microorganisms can survive. The efficiency of this sampler is
best for collecting particles less than 5 microns in
diameter.

In summary, it must be remembered that there exists
no one single air sampler that is 100 per cent efficient.
For extremely critical studies it is recommended that
two or three types be used side by side and that the
evaluation of a bacteriological air sample be based on
two or three different types of growth media in the
laboratory. In practice, however, this approach is un-
economical as well as definitely disadvantageous and
frequently hopeless, as the results may be so unrelated
and confusing that further studies would lead only to
the complete renunciation of all sampling methods together with a furious abnegation of bacteriology and
what it stands for. The novice must acquaint himself
not only with the operational methods but also with
the merits of each individual air sampling technique,
and even the experienced operator should not forget that
different methods give different results, and that the
sample to be evaluated may not represent a typical collection of microorganisms or particles in the air. There
is an air sampler available to test practically any

known conditions, but in order to select the proper air
sampling device for a study one must have a clear con-
ception of the type of information sought and of the
type of information a particular air sampling device
will give. It would be completely useless to publish
accurate figures of bacterial air contamination for,
let us say, one "clean room", without mentioning the
method of sampling and the type of information sought.
Similarly, at the present time it would be great folly
to standardize requirements for "clean rooms" on a
nation-wide scale; the state of affairs in the fields
of air bacteriology and contamination control is so
dynamic, and the innovations so frequent, that a flexi-
ble guide would be of more use than fixed requirements.
Each type of industry concerned with air contamination
should standardize and control contamination limits
within their own particular environment and to suit
their needs.

SUMMARY   OF   EVALUATION   OF   SAMPLERS

Gravitational settling. Not suited for immediate
quantitative evaluation, but satisfactory for studying
long-term trends in quantitation, typing, and sizing of
non-modified particles of large size.

Filtration. Not recommended for viability studies
of growing (vegetative) cells, unless microbial proce-
dures of rapid washing and plating of the collected
sample are immediately available. Not suggested for
long sampling times because of the tendency of organisms
exposed to air currents to dry out.

Centrifugal deposition. Gives good sampling efficiency with low concentrations of contamination, but
with samples that contain a high concentration of viable
particles, quantitation becomes problematic. Some devices are useful also in particle sizing.

Electrostatic precipitation. Well suited for high
sampling rates, but not for high concentrations of contamination. Viability results are good with nutrient
agar plates. Careful adjustment and expert maintenance
are needed.

Semi-solid and solid surface impaction. Devices
with agar impaction surfaces are excellent for viability
studies, particle sizing, and aerodynamic evaluation of
contamination. Usually recommended for high-volume

sampling. Well suited for absolute quantitation and time-concentration studies of particles. Paper-tape samplers are only satisfactory in the relative evaluation of non-biological contamination of air.

Liquid (capillary) impinging. Extremely favourable for quantitation of all particle sizes. Viability excellent even with high-volume sampling, but breaking up of clumps and the death of some susceptible vegetative cells at extremely high sampling velocities occur frequently.

COMMERCIAL   SOURCES   OF   SAMPLERS   MENTIONED

Gravitational Samplers
Petri plates are available from any general scientific supply house. They may be made of glass or of plastic.

Filtration Samplers
Sponge and fibre filters are not available commercially in a sampling device.
Membrane filters can be obtained from Gelman Instrument Co., Ann Arbor, Mich. or Millipore Filter Corp. (Canada), Montreal, P. Q.

Centrifugation Samplers
C. F. Casella & Co., Ltd. London, England.

Electrostatic Precipitation Samplers
General Electric Co., Cleveland, Ohio.

Slit Samplers
C. F. Casella & Co., Ltd., London, England.
Reynier & Sons, Chicago, Ill.

Drum Samplers and Multijet Monitors
Andersen Samplers, Provo, Utah.

Solid Surface Impactors
Gelman Instrument Co., Ann Arbor, Mich.

Liquid (Capillary) Impingers
Ace Glass, Inc., Vineland, N. J.
Millipore Filter Corp. (Canada), Montreal, P. Q.

LITERATURE   CITED

A. A. Andersen (1958), "New Sampler for the Collection, Sizing, and Enumeration of Viable Air-borne Particles," J. Bacteriol. 76: 471.

A. A. Andersen and M. R. Andersen (1961), "A Monitor for Air-borne Bacteria," Appl. Microbiol. 10: 181.

R. B. Bourdillon, O. M. Lidwell, and J. C. Thomas (1941), "A Slit Sampler for Collecting and Counting Air-borne Bacteria," J. Hyg. 41: 197.

R. Koch (1881), "Zur Untersuchung von pathogenen Organismen," Mitth. Kaiser. Gesundh. 1: 32.

M. Luckiesh, A. H. Taylor, and L. L. Holloday (1946), "Sampling Devices for Air-borne Bacteria," J. Bacteriol. 52: 55.

R. C. Marsh, W. J. Whitefield, and I. M. Kodel (1962), "Dry Slide Technique," Air Eng. 4: 44.

GENERAL REFERENCES

H. G. Dubuy, A. Hollaender, and M. D. Lackey (1945),
   "Comparative Studies of Sampling Devices for
   Air-borne Microorganisms," Publ. Health Repts.,
   Supp. 184.

A. J. Kluyver and J. Visser (1950), "The Determination
   of Microorganisms in Air," Ant. v. Leeuwenhoek,
   16: 299.

W. H. Rodebush (1950), "General Properties of Aerosols,"
   p. 60 of Handbook of Aerosols (Washington, D. C.:
   Atomic Energy Commission, U. S. Government Printing Office).

T. Rosebury (1947), Experimental Air-borne Infection,
   (Baltimore: Williams and Wilkins Co.).

H. W. Wolf et al. (1959), Sampling Microbiological
   Aerosols, Publ. Health Monograph No. 60 (Washington, D. C.:U. S. Government Printing Office).